Staying Healthy

Tips, Techniques and Diet

Suggestions for Heart Patients

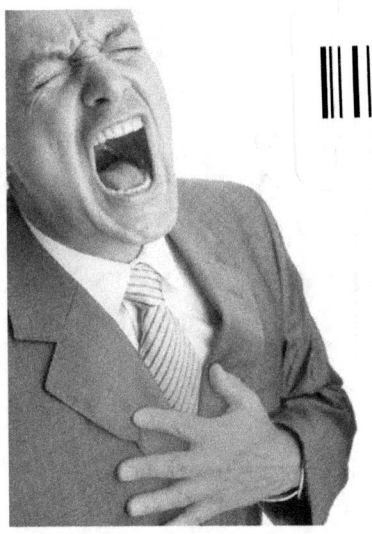

I0450185

Dueep J. Singh

Mendon Cottage Books

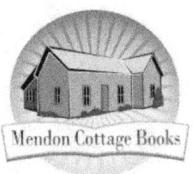

JD-Biz Publishing

All Rights Reserved.

No part of this publication may be reproduced in any form or by any means, including scanning, photocopying, or otherwise without prior written permission from JD-Biz Corp Copyright © 2014

All Images Licensed by Fotolia and 123RF.

Disclaimer

The information is this book is provided for informational purposes only. It is not intended to be used and medical advice or a substitute for proper medical treatment by a qualified health care provider. The information is believed to be accurate as presented based on research by the author.

The contents have not been evaluated by the U.S. Food and Drug Administration or any other Government or Health Organization and the contents in this book are not to be used to treat cure or prevent disease.

The author or publisher is not responsible for the use or safety of any diet, procedure or treatment mentioned in this book. The author or publisher is not responsible for errors or omissions that may exist.

Warning

The Book is for informational purposes only and before taking on any diet, treatment or medical procedure, it is recommended to consult with your primary health care provider.

Check out some of the other Healthy Gardening Series books at Amazon.com

Gardening Series on Amazon

Check out some of the other Health Learning Series books at Amazon.com

Health Learning Series on Amazon

Table of Contents

Introduction

One of the main reasons why I decided to write this book is because while doing research on heart ailments and natural ways in which to keep healthy, I found out some terrible statistics, which are not going to be told to you by your friendly neighborhood cardiologist.

Did you know that about 24.1 million people in the USA, alone suffer from heart disease? I thought that that was a terrible number, till I found that the statistics of Asian countries like India [60 million!] and China statistics were even more.

One out of every four people in Tasmania suffered from heart disease, and high blood pressure. They hold the world record for the most number of people suffering from heart disease. That was surprising, because I was under the impression that this could possibly have been the prerogative of those European countries, like Denmark, Sweden, and Norway, where food eaten every day was still in Emperor sized helpings, especially in the form of smorgasbords and jumbo sized sandwiches.

But then here are some reasons why heart disease statistics in these particular countries is comparatively low. First of all, they have a very healthy genetic background. Next, they believe in lots of exercise and do not bother much about sedentary lifestyles. These people are fit and fine because they cycle to work.

On the other hand, many people were slowly and steadily developing heart diseases all over the world today do so because of bad diet. Also, a paucity of antioxidants like vitamins A, C and E in your diet, as well as an excess of cholesterol and triglycerides are definitely major contributing factors for possible heart disease.

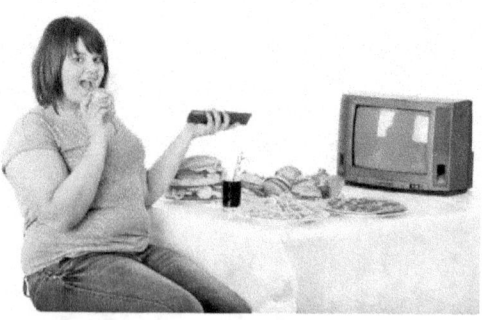

An unrestricted diet is going to have you more prone to heart disease.
Staying Healthy – Tips and Techniques For Heart Patients

Why Do so Many People Suffer from Heart Disease?

Having a cardiologist cousin, with his own 30 bed multi-specialty hospital, I spent a lot of time learning more about heart patients and heart diseases, through observation. I may not have a Medical Degree, but there are some things, which I noticed, and which may not have been told to you by a cardiologist.

Some of the major factors which lead to heart disease is the traditional oil based diet still being followed in a large number of countries, even though lifestyle circumstances have changed drastically during the latter half of the 20th century and the 21st century. We enjoy using a lot of cream, milk products, oil, and other items in our diet, because according to us, a dish is not tasty, unless it is butter-based or milk-based.

This mindset is responsible for the increasing number of heart patients all over the world today. Also, a sedentary lifestyle, as well as stress and strain can also have a direct effect upon your heart.

Naturally, I asked my brother about why cardiologists dealing with heart diseases do not bother much about educating their patients about heart disease and its treatment? His answer was that the world was made up of people who did not want to learn and people who would not bother about advice given. They would rather have their cardiologist cure them. That is why a number of cardio surgeons and doctors decided to take full advantage of this ignorance.

That is the reason why you are seeing so many coronary care units and multi-speciality heart disease hospitals blooming all over the landscape. Many of the cardiac surgeons are minting millions, by doing angioplasties and bypass surgeries. That is because the patients are under the impression that these are the only ways in which their heart disease problem can be solved.

This is so not true. These comparative modern measures are definitely not the only resorts possible for a person suffering from heart disease. You can prevent as well as reduce it with the help of your diet, your lifestyle and other easy to implement points given to you further on.

In fact, most of these surgical measures are just temporary measures. Many of these patients go back to those hospitals after a couple of years, thus enriching the doctors yet once again.

Staying Healthy – Tips and Techniques For Heart Patients

As prevention is better than cure, you need to know all about the causative factors of heart diseases, and Ways and Means in which you can prevent the disease from growing.

Did you know that it is possible to reverse heart disease? We have Dr. Dean Michael Ornish to thank for that particular knowledge, which is based on ancient knowledge and commonsense. http://www.webmd.com/diet/ornish-diet-what-it-is reviews his diet plans but he is just speaking of a way of life which has been followed by millions of people all over the world down the millenniums and all over the globe.

So for all those people who want to know more about the heart and heart diseases, here is some general information about the heart its functions and what is heart disease.

Some "Hearty" Information

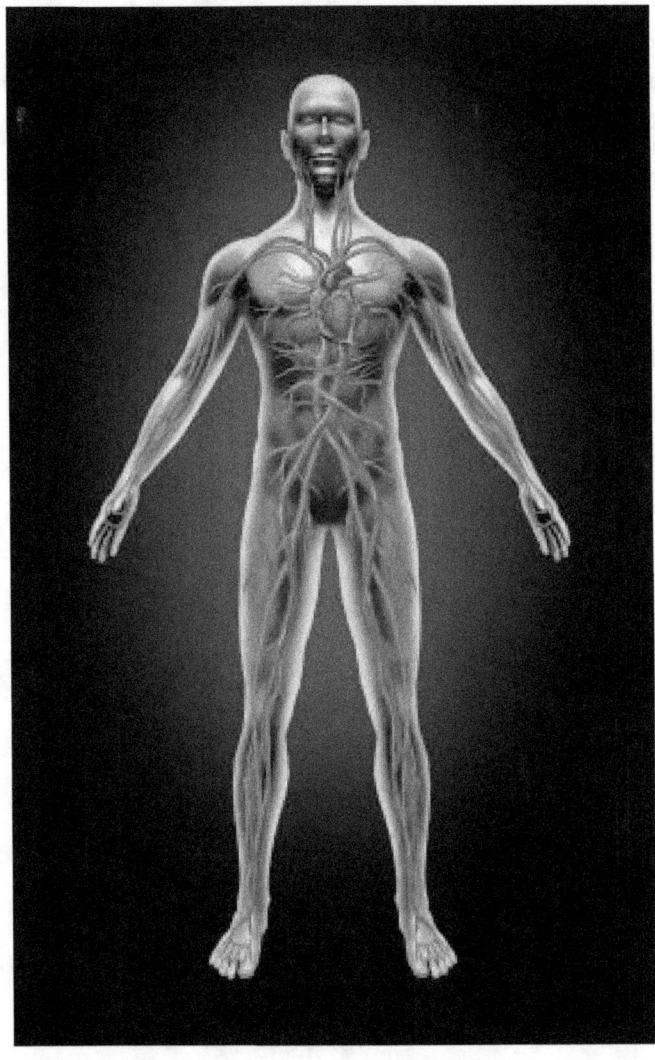

The human heart is a small, powerful muscular organ, somewhat centered and tilted to the left side of your chest. It weighs about 350 g, yet is powerful enough to supply blood through pumping throughout the body. This blood is going to supply oxygen and nutrients to the whole body and to all the cells in it. This circulated free system also carries vitamins and minerals to all the cells of the body without which the body cannot function properly and, naturally, in a healthy manner and well.

It also helps in the carrying or pulling of the blood back to the heart and sending that same blood to the lungs for an oxygen refill.
Staying Healthy – Tips and Techniques For Heart Patients

Neuro– Chemicals and hormones are also ferried from one part of the body to another through this blood circulation, pumped by the heart.

It also helps in taking the waste materials to the kidneys for purification. The wastes are removed by the body's natural eliminating system after the kidney extracts all the harmful waste and toxins from the blood.

What Is Heart Disease –

Angina Pectoris

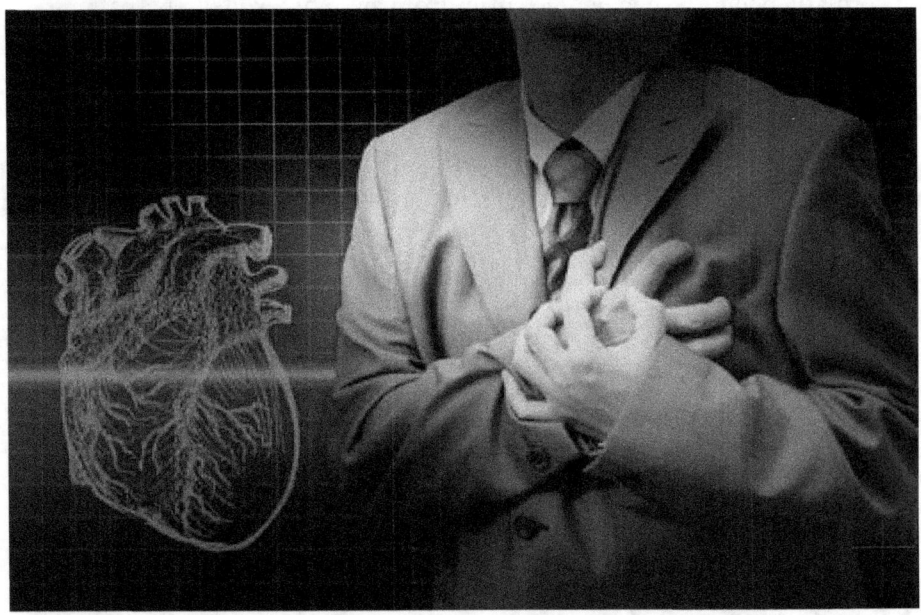

The heart being a vulnerable part of the normal body is subject to a number of ailments, like other parts of the body. Some of the factors contributing to coronary heart disease can be attributed to your genetic makeup. If your family is prone to heart disease, there is a chance that you are also going to suffer from it sometime or the other in your life. Also, your lifestyle is definitely going to have a positive or negative effect on your future good or ill functioning of this very important pumping machine.

Believe it or not, it takes anywhere between 3 to 5 years for a completely healthy person to become vulnerable to heart disease. That is when he starts taking the wrong sort of food, including fatty food and cholesterol laden food. Let us say, this is one of the reasons I can consider myself a possible future victim of heart disease.

Sitting in front of the computer from 9 to 5 – as do so many of us –, with absolutely no exercise, eating whatever junk food is placed before us, or just skipping meals, these are some of the contributing factors which can have you developing blockages in your heart tubes.

Angina is a sensation of pain or heaviness in the left side of your chest, which radiates to the left arm and is associated with a choking sensation, sweating and breathlessness.

This normally occurs, when people suffer from anxiety, excitement, bathing in very cold water, walking, climbing stairs, or during any activity which causes physical and mental stress. People eating heavy meals may suffer such discomfort after a little bit of exertion on their parts. This discomfort can be relieved by resting, or taking a nitroglycerin tablet placed below the tongue. In most cases, this pain is not excruciating and does not cause discomfort for a long time. But if these two occur simultaneously, you can consider that to be a heart attack, which is known medically as **myocardial infarction Or Coronary Thrombosis**.

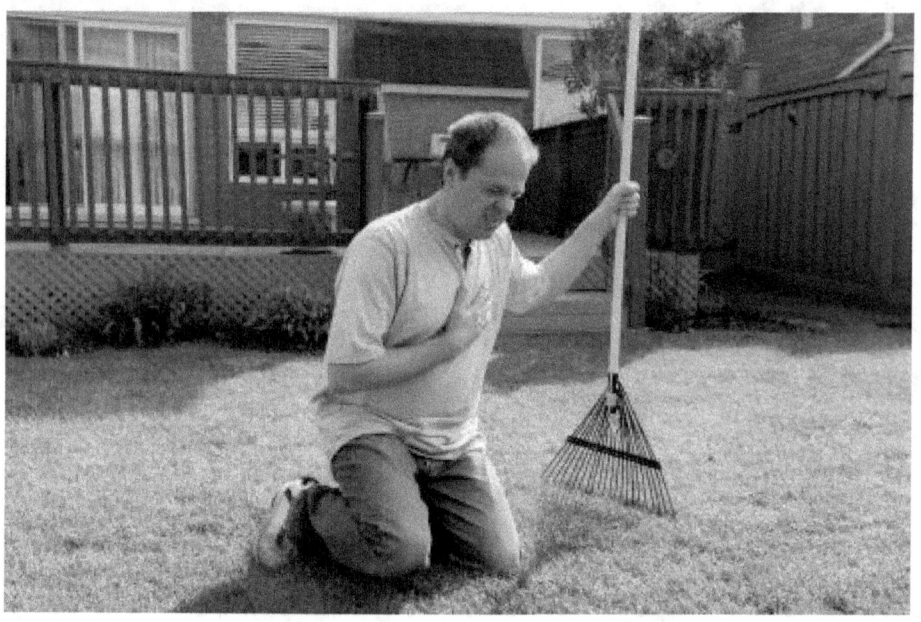

The starting point is always going to be zero. With more and more layers of fat piling up in your arteries, you are going to have artery blockage up to 70%. You find yourself panting, sweating, and your general state of good health going downhill really fast. So you decide to ask your doctor for a thorough checkup. He immediately diagnoses heart disease.

Your immediate reaction is – "that is so not true. I am healthy and hearty, it is just I put on a little bit of weight, I do not suffer from any heart disease. There is absolutely no chance that I could ever be prone to such a possibility of my heart suffering from any such ailment."

Staying Healthy – Tips and Techniques For Heart Patients

But alas, the proof of the pudding is in the eating and all the rich puddings eaten for lunch every day, have finally taken their toll. And so we find ourselves prey to heart problems.

CHD/IHD

Heart disease is any disease, which is caused by the accumulation of cholesterol or fats in the arteries. These arteries are the blood carrying tubes in the walls of the heart. 95% of heart ailments are caused because of this accumulation. This is because there has been an obstruction of blood flow to the heart, causing a heart attack or a possible stroke.

This blockage of heart disease is normally referred to a CHD Or Coronary Heart Disease. You may know it as angina pectoris. It normally shows up as a pain on the left side of the chest, radiating to your left arm. 80% of the people suffer from this form of heart trouble – Angina. It is also known as ischemia, which is also known as shortness of oxygen. You may also find doctors referring to CHD as Ischemic heart disease or IHD.

How do you recognize that you are suffering from a heart attack?

Heart Attack Symptoms

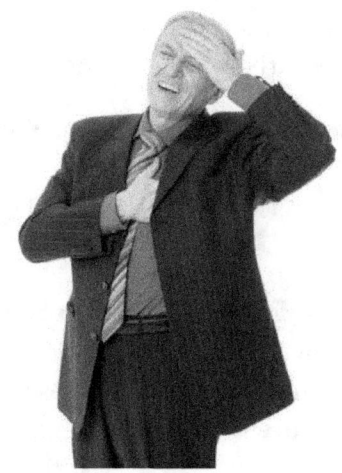

Angina Pain can be anywhere from mild to severe, but the pain caused due to heart attack is extremely severe. It usually occurs in the center of the chest and radiates to the left arm, but at times it even radiates to the shoulders, right arm or the lower jaw. This pain usually lasts for five – 10 minutes

The patient is also going to suffer from shortness of breath, sweating, nausea, fainting and dizziness. Other symptoms include weakness, or choking sensation in your throat, heaviness or tightness in the chest or the upper portion of the abdomen. You may find yourself suffering from this pain, especially after heavy meals.

When Can Heart Attacks Occur?

A heart attack can often occur after a heavy meal full of fat, after sudden displays of anger, excessive sorrow, shock or grief, or even excessive stress. These attacks occur more frequently early in the morning.

This angina occurs when the arterial blockage is more than 70%. A heart attack is going to occur due to 100% blockage in any of the coronary arteries or their branches. The heart muscles are completely deprived of oxygen and blood supply, which leads to death.

The severity of a heart attack is going to depend on how much of heart muscle is involved. Many patients survive a mild heart attack, when only 5 to 10% of the area is involved. However, if the dead heart muscles are more than 30 to 40%, this attack is considered to be severe. If not managed properly and immediately, it can be fatal in many cases.

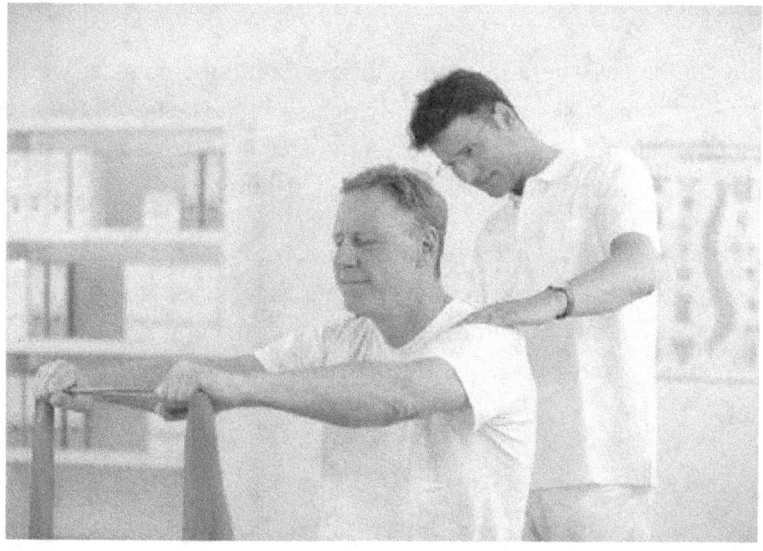

Regular medical checkups can help you monitor the state of your health as well as give you an indication of potential heart problems.

Controllable and Uncontrollable Risk Factors

There are some factors which contribute to heart disease and which cannot be controlled, – these include gender, age and heredity. These conditions are reasons or the risk factors, which aggravate or lead to the deposit of fat and cholesterol in the coronary arteries and lead to possible heart problems and heart attacks. The uncontrollable risk factors cannot be altered. The controllable risk factors can be controlled and modified to prevent coronary heart disease.

These factors include high levels of blood cholesterol and triglycerides, diabetes, stress, obesity, lack of physical activity, thanks to a sedentary lifestyle, alcohol and tobacco consumption and a bad diet, with lots of fat and lack of antioxidants.

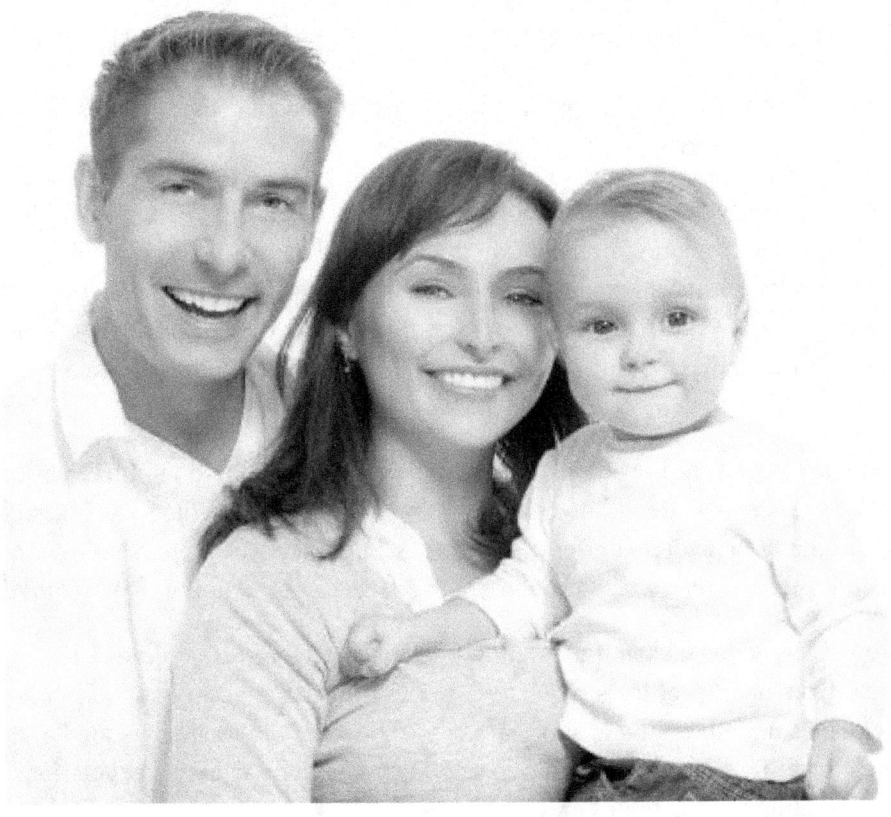

A healthy genetic background means less chance of heart trouble in the future for this healthy youngster.

Best Diet

I was talking to my father about how many people suffer from heart problems in the area in which he was born, and he said that such cases were quite limited. That was because people ate healthy meals, with less of meat and less of oil, worked terribly hard throughout the day and night, and as far as possible, tried to live lives without too much of stress and tension. So here were some items which were part of his diet as a youngster – raisins and dates, plenty of green vegetables, especially, green leafy vegetables like spinach, cabbages, lettuces, cucumber, and celery.

In fact, salads, made up of lettuce leaves are still being eaten by the low family, every day, especially as the lettuce leaves are low in calories. There are also helpful as part of weight reducing diets as long as they are not coated in fatty salad dressing, such as mayonnaise or olive oil based salad dressing. Thanks to the large amount of Beta carotene in lettuce leaves, you can stop diseases like atherosclerosis occurring.

Antioxidants are natural food agents which oppose oxidation, you can consider oxidation to be a damaging process which causes the degeneration of healthy tissue. When cholesterol is oxidized it builds up deposits, which cause blockages in the heart tissue. Antioxidants in your food, are going to be foodstuffs which are rich in vitamin A, C and E. Mineral antioxidants are calcium, zinc and selenium.

Natural fiber is present in fruit, as well as in vegetables. They do not have any calories, because they are going to increase the bulk content in the food ingested and are going to be excreted after digestion. All the fat particles present in your food can be considered to be "meshed" in this fiber, and are going to be removed.

Try a completely vegetarian diet along with fruit diet. Even if you are not suffering from heart problems, you are going to find a change in your health. It is no wonder that millenniums ago that the wise men of the East advocated a complete meat free diet for human beings. They knew the value of vegetarian meals consisting of vegetables and fruits.

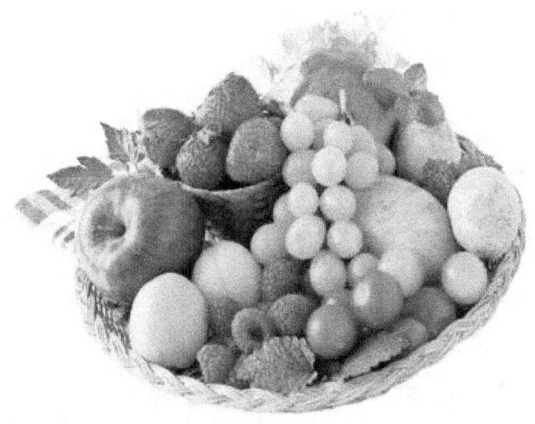

A Totally No – Oil Diet

I asked my cardiologist cousin, why he being a cardiologist – and incidentally a potential victim of heart attack, which was inherited genetically – continued eating a diet rich in oil and butter, and he said that this is a risk factor, which unfortunately cannot be controlled by a large number of people in Asia. Eating good food and rich food, and in large and lavish quantities is a part of many lifestyles. Ceremonies, festivals, social gatherings and other occasions are going to contribute to your intake of oil, because most of the food stuffs are going to be cooked in either oil or clarified butter. So even though he suffered from a heart attack at the age of 45, he cannot resist eating a diet rich in fats and oils.

If doctors can behave in such a childish manner, we cannot expect human beings like you and I to behave in a more responsible manner. That is a fact of life, because we would rather be led into temptation and let tomorrow take care of itself, when confronted with appetizing food which we are prevented from enjoying.

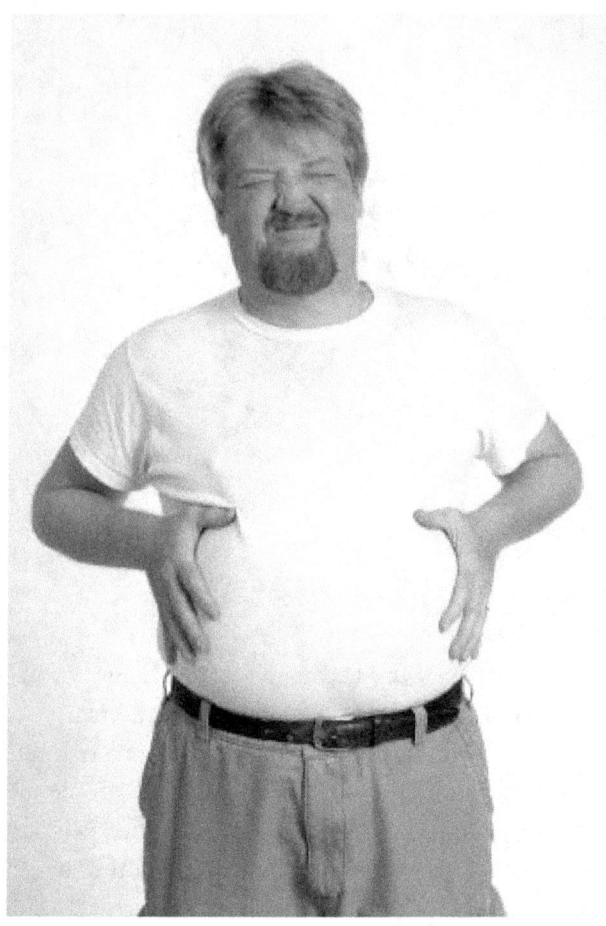

Obesity and a diet which has not been controlled is one of the main contributing factors for heart disease.

If you have the willpower and the dedication to follow a no oil rule, you are going to prevent obesity, as well as potential heart diseases. Remember that fat takes a longer time to get digested so it stores itself in the body. Muscles thus find themselves covered with a layer of fat. This leads to obesity.

When there is excess of fat in the blood, it settles down in the arteries and creates blockages. So when there is so much fat in the body, adding more fat content to the already present layer of cellulite is going to cause you potential heart problems in the future.

All oils are hundred percent fats. A major constituent of all these oils are triglycerides. The two fats depositing in the insides of the tubes supplying the blood to the heart are triglycerides and cholesterol. The moment you take an excess amount of oil, your blood level of triglyceride is going to increase. The moment the blood level of a triglyceride exceeds a particular level, – about 130 MG/DL –, the chances of more blockages being formed increase. Therefore, any sort of oil is bad for the heart and should be avoided diligently.

Butter is one item which is definitely not going to be a part of your diet, especially if you suffer from obesity or you are a potential heart patient. Butter is nothing but hundred percent fat. It is formed by churning cream, which is fat.

Butter is also a milk product, which has a high level of cholesterol in it. Cholesterol is the most well-known causative agents for blockages and heart diseases.

Long, long ago, our ancestors used to eat a diet full of cream, milk and butter and keep healthy. But then they did not have sedentary lifestyles. They worked hard outdoors, from morning till late at night so the butter never had a chance to accumulate and settle in their arteries. That is not the case today. Our sedentary lifestyles make it impossible for a large number of us to burn up extra calories. So no butter.

This no oil rule also unfortunately includes no dry fruit and nuts. So you cannot eat almonds, pistachios, walnuts and groundnuts, either. They are rich in fat.

Home remedies for obesity:

- Honey
- Lemon
- Plain water
- Ginger
- Apple cider vinegar
- Carrot juice
- Pepper
- Salads

Fish Oil In Your Diet

I was shocked to see a number of supposed medical authorities on the Internet telling you that fish oil is good for heart patients because of its omega-3 content. **This is totally false**. Fish oil is an animal source product. Any oil from a natural animal source has lots of cholesterol. Cholesterol is the primary cause of blockage. QED. So anybody who can add one plus one should understand that fish oil, along with other animal source products should be avoided diligently by people who suffer from heart problems.

On the other hand, pulses and cereals are plant sources of omega-3 fatty acids. These are definitely not harmful for your heart, so they should be taken in large quantities to give your heart healthy.

In the same manner anybody telling you that some particular brand of marketed oil is cholesterol free and heart friendly is misguiding you. These labels are marketing strategies, especially when they tell you that they are going to reduce cholesterol levels. Remember that cholesterol is present only in animal products. Since all these oils are obtained from plant products, especially sunflowers, where do you suppose cholesterol comes in here? However, these oils have triglycerides which are equally responsible in causing blockages in your heart.

So the next time you are tempted to pour lots of sunflower oil on your salad, because hey, the marketing company says that it helps reduce cholesterol levels, remember that this oil is equally responsible for causing arterial buildup and heart blockages.

Lowering Your Triglyceride Level

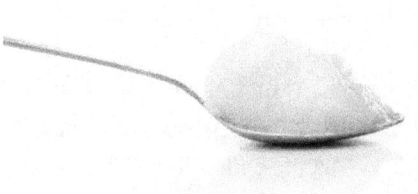

You may consider the addition of all this butter to be essential to a flavorful diet, but it is one of the main reasons why you may suffer from potential heart disease in the future.

Apart from reducing the oil intake because they are nothing but triglycerides, you can also reduce your intake of sugar and other simple carbohydrates. This is going to include white rice, white flour and alcohol, which is converted by the body into sugar. The simple carbohydrates are absorbed very quickly, causing the blood glucose level to rise quickly. In response to this, the pancreas secretes insulin in order to lower the blood sugar to a normal range. This is good. Nevertheless, insulin also accelerates the conversion of the calories in your body into triglycerides.

Whole foods, which are also known as complex carbohydrates include grains, beans, fruit, vegetables, whole wheat flour and brown rice in its natural form. These foods are rich in fiber. The absorption of food gets slowed down with fiber. So that means you are not going to see a rapid rise in blood glucose and excessive insulin production. Besides this, you find yourself more energetic throughout the day.

Some food items which have oil content less than 1 g per hundred grams include corn, green leafy vegetables, mint, potato, pumpkins, apples, guavas and musk melon. So add these to your diet. Yes, hundred grams of potato, boiled or roasted and not fried.

Oatmeal As a Healthy Cereal

I wondered why more and more people are not eating oatmeal as a natural surreal, especially as a lunch dish. It is extremely good for heart patients. That is when it is in its unrefined form. Oatmeal bran is an important source of fiber, which helps to control the level of cholesterol in your body.

Oatmeal has oat germ, which is more nutritious than wheat bran. That is why Scottish oatmeal porridge is one of the main reasons why the Scotch do not suffer much from heart ailments. These oats are also helpful in stabilizing the blood sugar and antioxidant activity. Someone told me that people suffering from nicotine cravings can get rid of them by just eating some oatmeal. So the next time you want to reach for a cigarette, you may want to substitute some healthy oatmeal instead.

In the same manner, corn, with its fiber content helps in binding the cholesterol and lowering its level in the blood. You can either have corn on the cob or as cornbread or cornflakes.

White Bread or Brown?

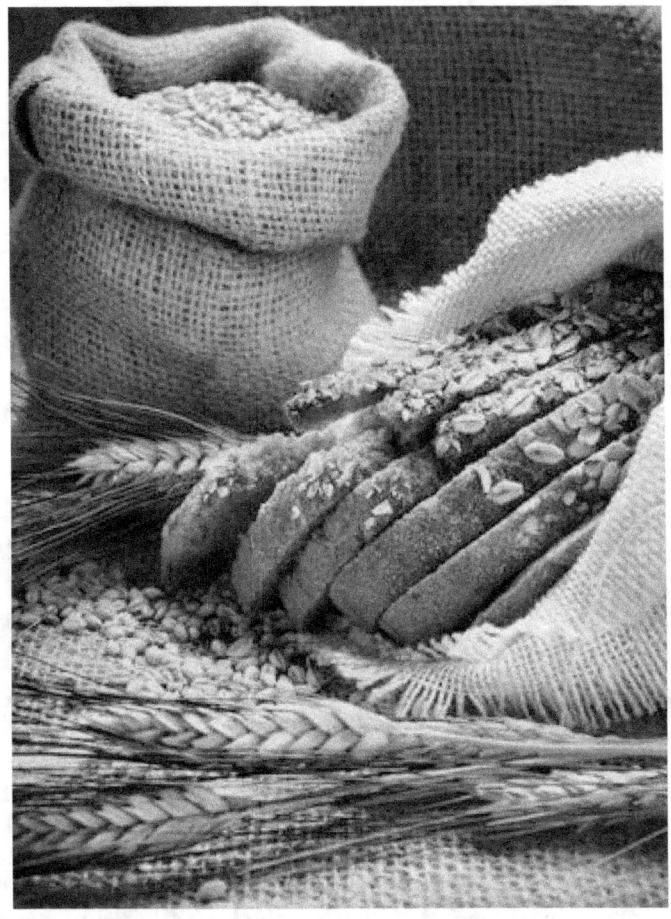

White bread is made up of refined flour. This has low fiber content. Brown bread is made up of whole wheat with a higher fiber content. So, because brown bread has a good amount of B complex vitamins and is rich in fibers, you may want to add that to your diet, instead of white bread. Brown bread is also excellent for diabetics.

On the other hand, white bread is made up of flour which has been built from the inner part of the wheat grain after the husk has been removed. All the good nutritive portions of flour are thus removed and additives like emulsifiers and preservatives are added to this popular marketed sandwich bread. Good to look at, not so good to eat.

If you cannot do without macaroni or pasta, make sure that you add a lot of vegetables to help reduce the refined flour content.

What about Soybean?

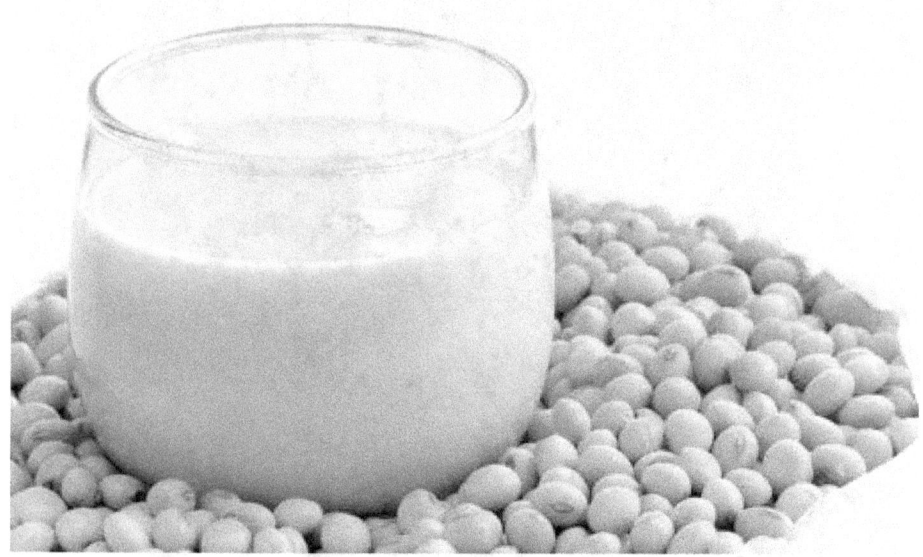

Soybean is considered to be the king of pulses in many parts of Asia. It is a rich source of protein. Find in these studies in the USA have proven that have been protein reduces cholesterol levels. It also has the high fiber content, which reduces blood sugar levels. When the cholesterol levels are low, there are less chances of blockages and further heart disease occurring.

The popular Japanese food item – tofu is made up of soybean. This is made by grinding cooked soybeans to produce soybean milk which is then solidified with a mineral coagulant , like calcium sulfate. This is high in protein, very low in saturated fats and cholesterol free, and that is why so many people eat plenty of tofu for lunch, all over the world. This is naturally bland and you can use it in both sweet and savory dishes.

Tofu is high in protein and low in saturated fats. It is also a good source of calcium and vitamin E. However, remember that soybean in excess is not advisable. That is because this is very high in protein and consumption of a high amount of proteins is going to affect the functioning of your kidneys. It also has
Staying Healthy – Tips and Techniques For Heart Patients

a high amount of fat which can lead to heart problems. That is why it should always be used after it has been processed and turned into tofu.

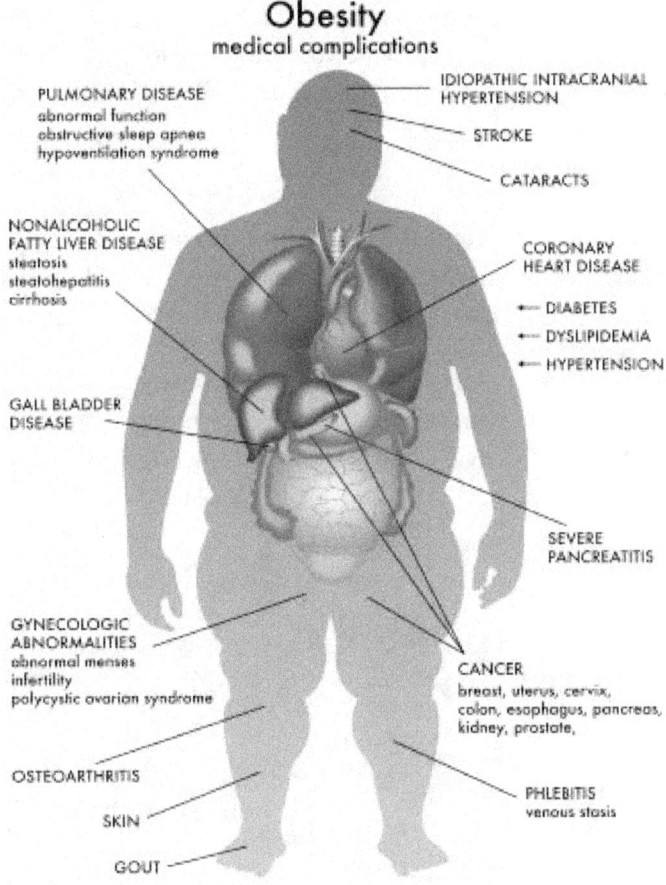

Apart from potential heart diseases, obesity is also the main culprit and factor causing many other diseases in your body.

So for all those people who are interested in the best food with which they can reduce weight, as well as keep their hearts healthy, I would suggest Sprouts.

They are good for the heart as they are rich in fiber and natural antioxidants like vitamins C and vitamin E. Sprouts also help in reducing weight.

How to Make Sprouts

Sprouts can be made from any beans type and variety, even though lentils like mung are the most popular traditional mediums for making this nutritious addition to your diet. To make sprouts, you are going to dip a clean piece of cloth in water and then wring it out. Take your choice of grains/pulses and spread them all over that wet and moist cloth. Cover the grains with another layer of wet and moist cloth.

Keep for 36 – 48 hours, making sure that the water content on the cloth remains ever present because after all these seeds are germinating. After 48 hours, you are going to get sprouted grains, which can be eaten in the morning with breakfast, or whenever required.

Do not fry them in oil. If you are a heart patient, you may want to just dry stirfry in a wok and sprinkle it all over your food or add to your salad.

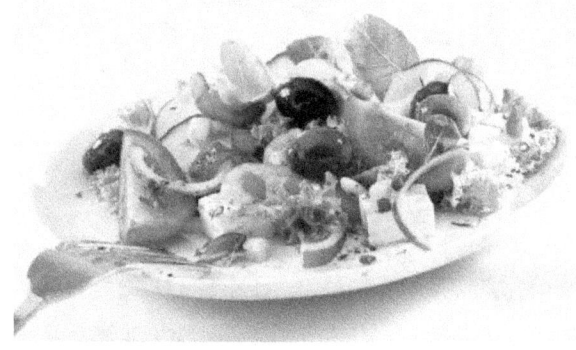

Try making salads a part of your daily diet. Sprouts can be added to these salads, and you can sprinkle some herbs on them to give them more taste and flavor. As you cannot use salad dressing because of the oil content, add some yogurt, which has been made by skimmed milk. Yogurt is basically pasteurized or homogenized milk in which a bacterial culture has been added. This is a useful source of calcium and phosphorus. It also contains necessary vitamins like B 2 and B12, which helped to replace valuable bacteria in your digestive system and which also helps in the boosting of the immunity system.

Salads can be taken throughout the day, and in whatever quantity you wish, as long as you do not smother them with mayonnaise or rich salad dressings. Just make sure that you are not underweight. If that is the case, you are going to tend to lose more weight. That is why salads are used for weight loss. That is because they provide a rich source of fiber and also provide more bulk to your diet. They also help eliminate the sugar and cholesterol present in your diet. Cauliflowers and radishes included in your salads may produce flatulence. So add some fenugreek seeds or aniseeds to the salad.

Many high-fiber yogurts are being marketed today as good cholesterol lowering food items. They have more soluble fiber added to them. I am not very certain about what that soluble fiber is [after all, it is a manufactured product and processed, and so I would not trust it –] so I would suggest that the yogurt you make at home should have skim milk as its manufacturing content.

Someone just asked me that he did not have access to toned and skimmed milk in his locality, but he knew about a farm near by, where he could get fresh milk. So would that be advisable? Well, taken from an Asiatic point of view, where people still get milk from their local milkmen, I would say that is all right, because those milk men are clever enough to remove the cream from the milk before selling it! And ain't that the truth.

But if you come up against honest milkmen, just remove the cream by boiling the milk and refrigerating it. After cooling for six hours, you are going to find a layer of cream on the surface. Remove the cream, boil the milk again and remove the second layer of cream. Now this milk can be called toned or skimmed milk and is good for drinking.

What, No Meat?

Now this is something up with most of us carnivorous beings will not put. The idea of our favorite juicy sausages, hamburgers, steaks, kidney pie and other meat products, which we enjoy so much being totally banned just because we suffer from heart problems is definitely not acceptable. This includes fish, red meat, chicken, lean meat, beef, pork and other meat products. You can take the white of an egg, which is rich in albumin and is more easily digested than the Yolk.

But that is the bitter truth because all organic meat products include lots of cholesterol and triglycerides. Even though beef has an excellent range of nutrients like iron, zinc and other valuable minerals, being rich in cholesterol means that you are going to be more prone to heart disease. Same thing goes for pork.

So your next response is – no meat and a restricted intake of milk products because milk is an animal product and has about four – 6% of fat in it, how are you going to make up for any sort of protein and mineral deficiency caused due to the paucity of these items in your diet?

Any sort of protein deficiency in your diet can be made up by eating lots of vegetarian foods like green leafy vegetables. These include spinach, fenugreek and other leafy plants. Beans and pulses like Mung, beans and milk products which are made of skimmed milk can compensate for any sort of protein loss caused by the removal of me from your daily diet. Along with that, you can eat mushrooms, sprouts, and whole grains like whole wheat, rice, etc..

Soya milk has no cholesterol, and Soya products actually lower your blood cholesterol levels. So if you get Soya milk easily, add that to your diet and make yogurt from it.

What about Tomatoes?

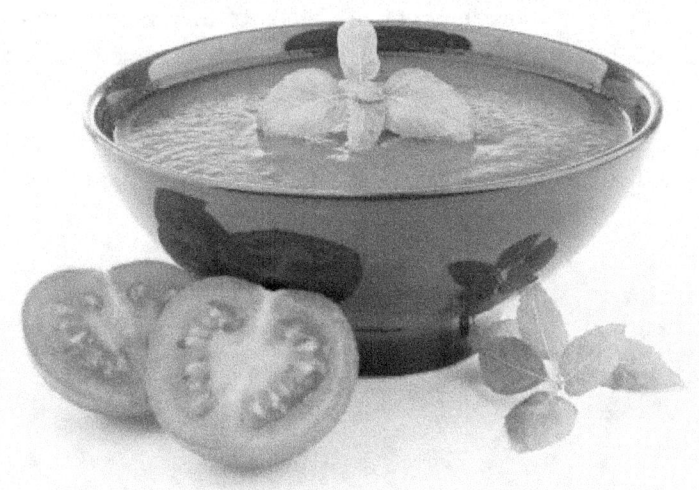

Tomatoes are considered to be good for the heart, because they contain nicotinic acid. This is believed to reduce cholesterol and vitamin K content in the tomatoes is an anti-hemorrhagic.

Tomatoes have long been used as an antiseptic, as well as a preventative food against infections for millenniums.

Lots of tomato juice drunk regularly means that you are going to have a natural blood purifier, getting into your system. It is also supposedly excellent for a therapeutic treatment of arthritis.

Conclusion

This book is full of tips and information about heart problems and how you can keep healthy through either preventing your heart from developing a heart problem or even getting more aggravated. Many of the tips are common sense tips which can be used by any newbie and which should have been told to you by your doctor.

So keep healthy,Live Long and Prosper!

Author Bio-

Dueep Jyot Singh is a Management and IT Professional who managed to gather Postgraduate qualifications in Management and English and Degrees in Science, French and Education while pursuing different enjoyable career options like being an hospital administrator, IT,SEO and HRD Database Manager/ trainer, movie , radio and TV scriptwriter, theatre artiste and public speaker, lecturer in French, Marketing and Advertising, ex-Editor of Hearts On Fire (now known as Solstice) Books Missouri USA, advice columnist and cartoonist, publisher and Aviation School trainer, ex- moderator on Medico.in, banker, student councilor ,travelogue writer … among other things!

One fine morning, she decided that she had enough of killing herself by Degrees and went back to her first love—writing. It's more enjoyable! She already has 48 published academic and 14 fiction- in- different- genre books under her belt.

When she is not designing websites or making Graphic design illustrations for clients , she is browsing through old bookshops hunting for treasures, of which she has an enviable collection – including R.L. Stevenson, O.Henry, Dornford Yates, Maurice Walsh, De Maupassant, Victor Hugo, Sapper, C.N. Williamson, "Bartimeus" and the crown of her collection- Dickens "The Old Curiosity Shop," and so on… Just call her "Renaissance Woman") - collecting herbal remedies, acting like Universal Helping Hand/Agony Aunt, or escaping to her dear mountains for a bit of exploring, collecting herbs and plants and trekking.

Our books are available at

1. Amazon.com
2. Barnes and Noble
3. Itunes
4. Kobo
5. Smashwords
6. Google Play Books

Check out some of the other JD-Biz Publishing books

Gardening Series on Amazon

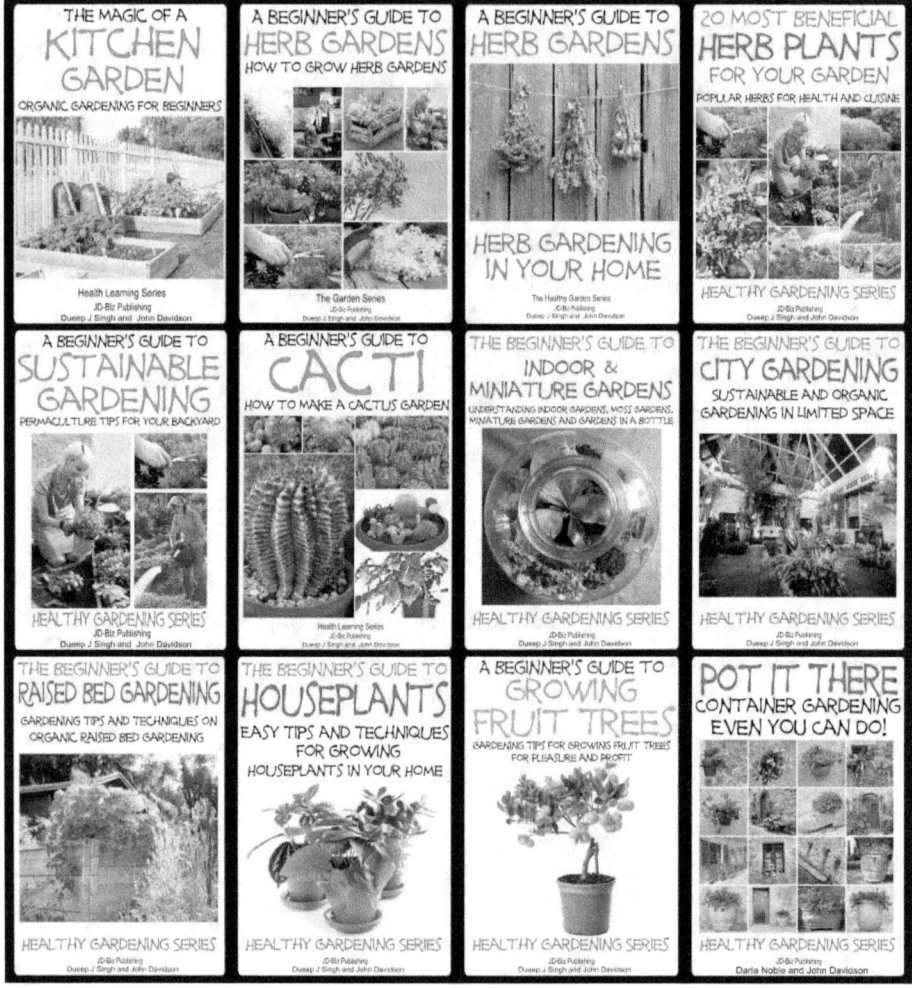

Staying Healthy – Tips and Techniques For Heart Patients

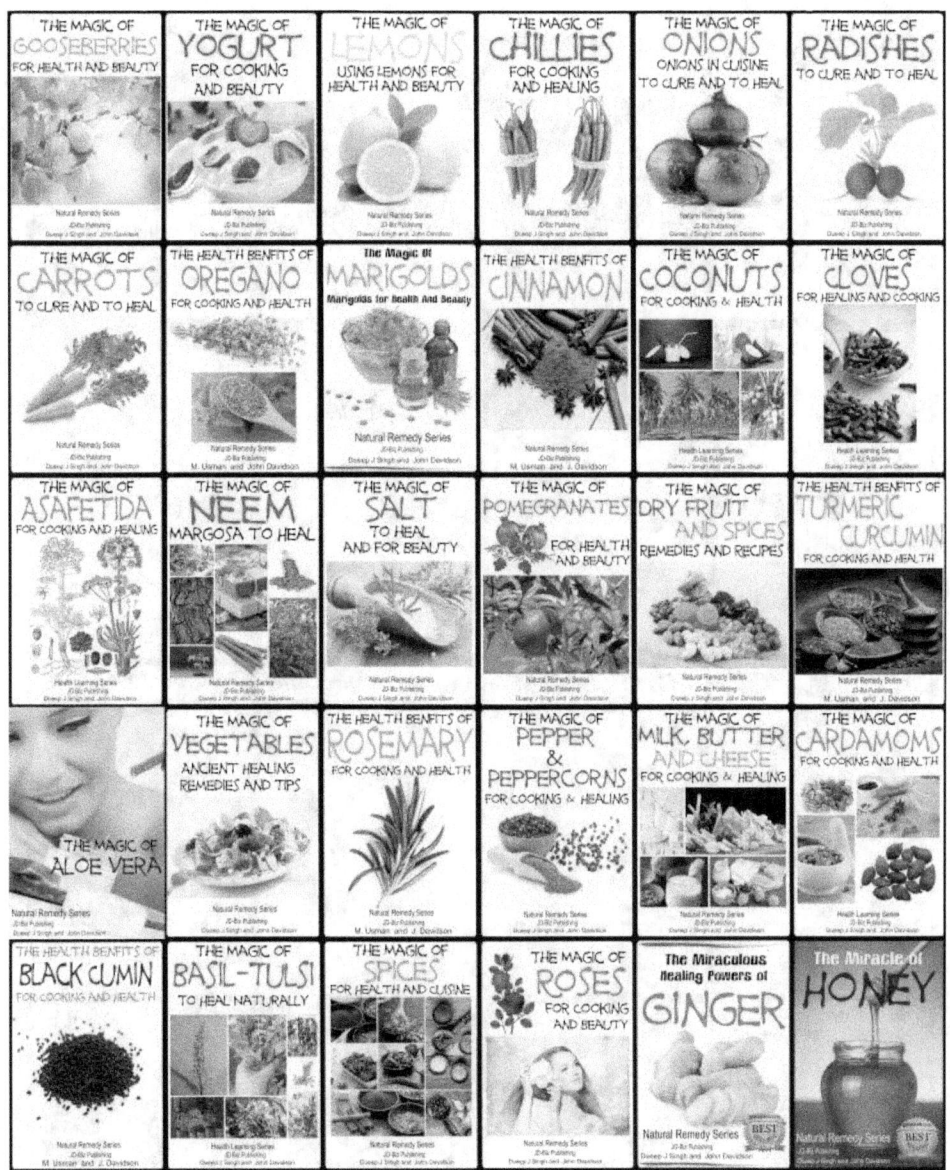

Staying Healthy – Tips and Techniques For Heart Patients

Country Life Books

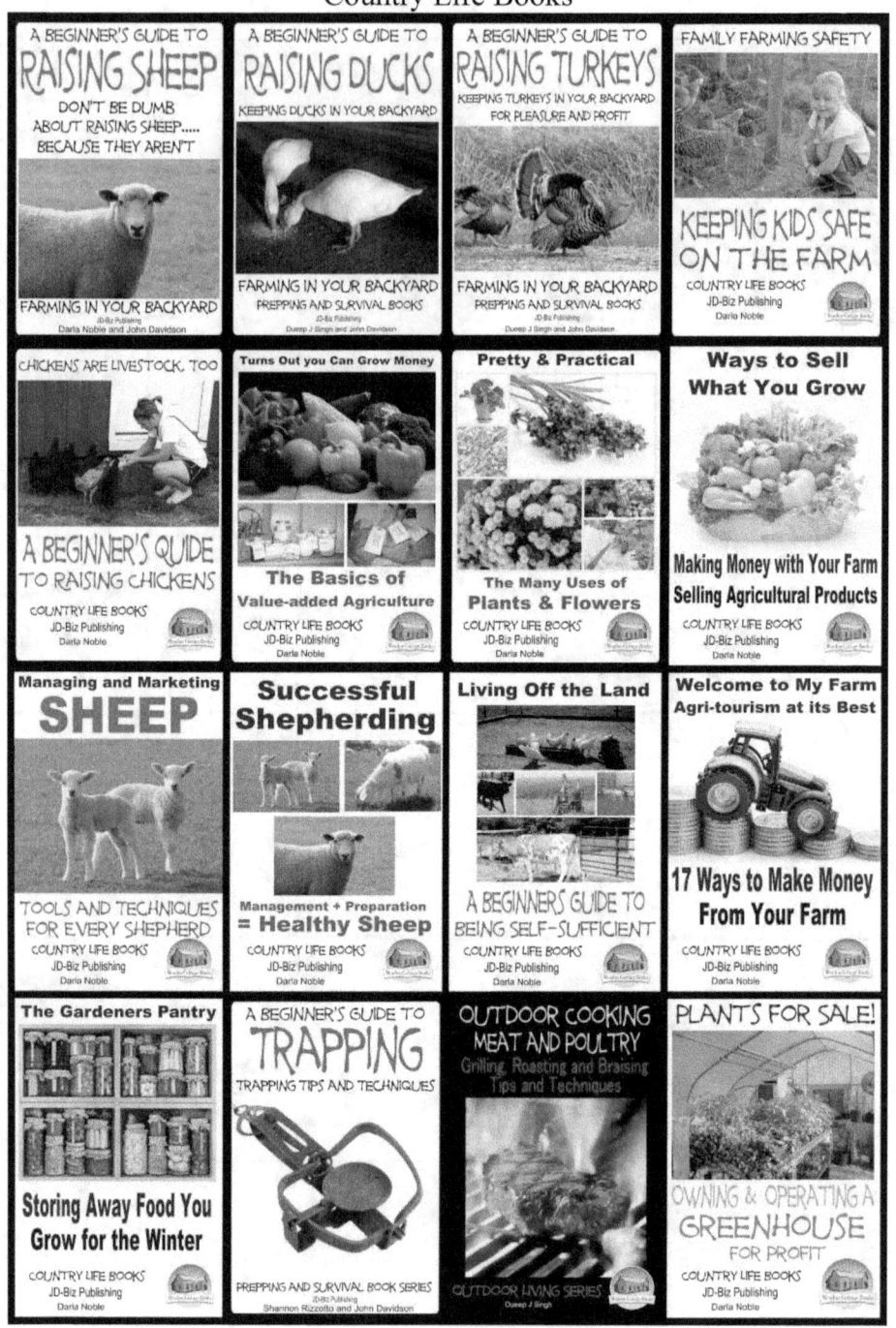

Staying Healthy – Tips and Techniques For Heart Patients

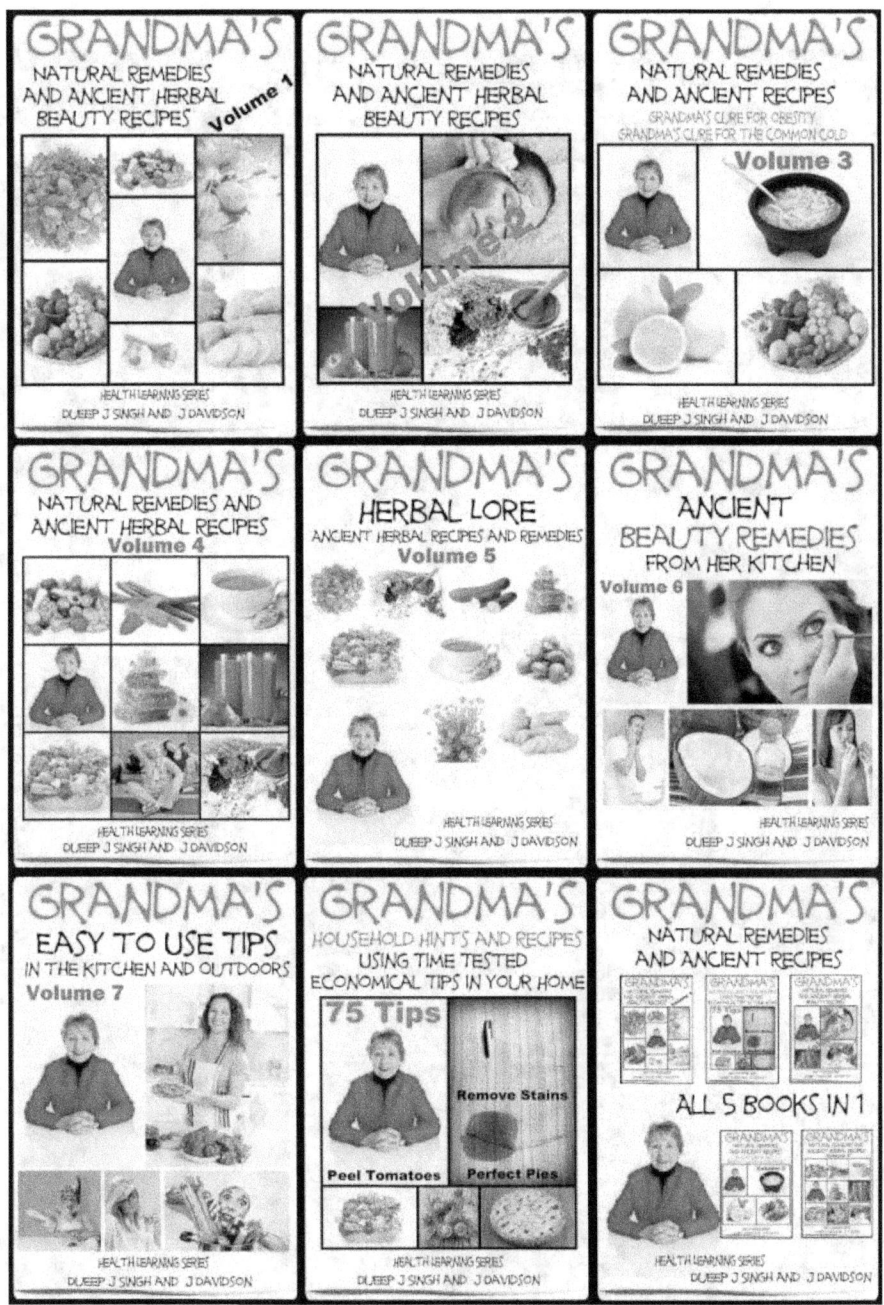

Staying Healthy – Tips and Techniques For Heart Patients

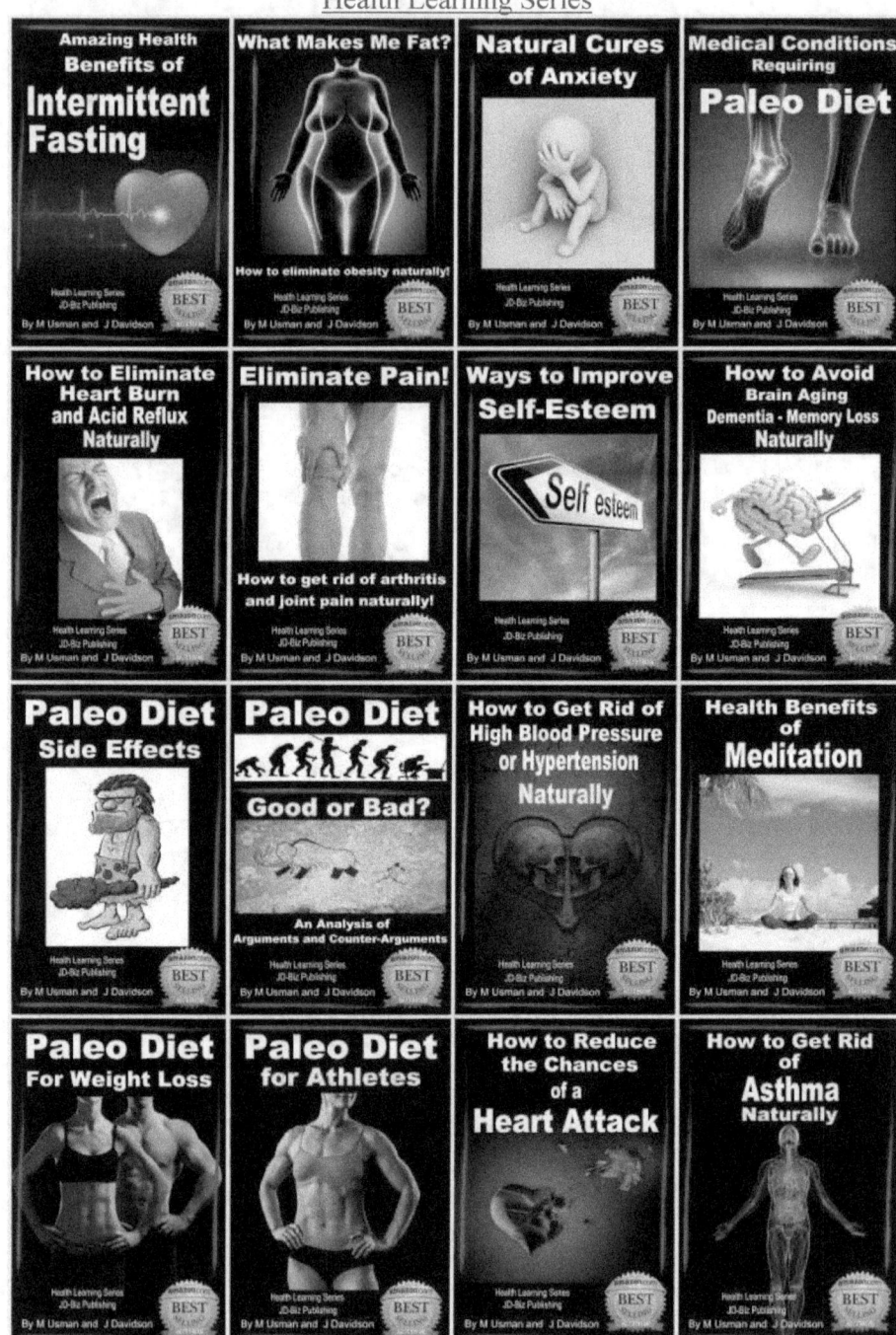

Staying Healthy – Tips and Techniques For Heart Patients

Amazing Animal Book Series

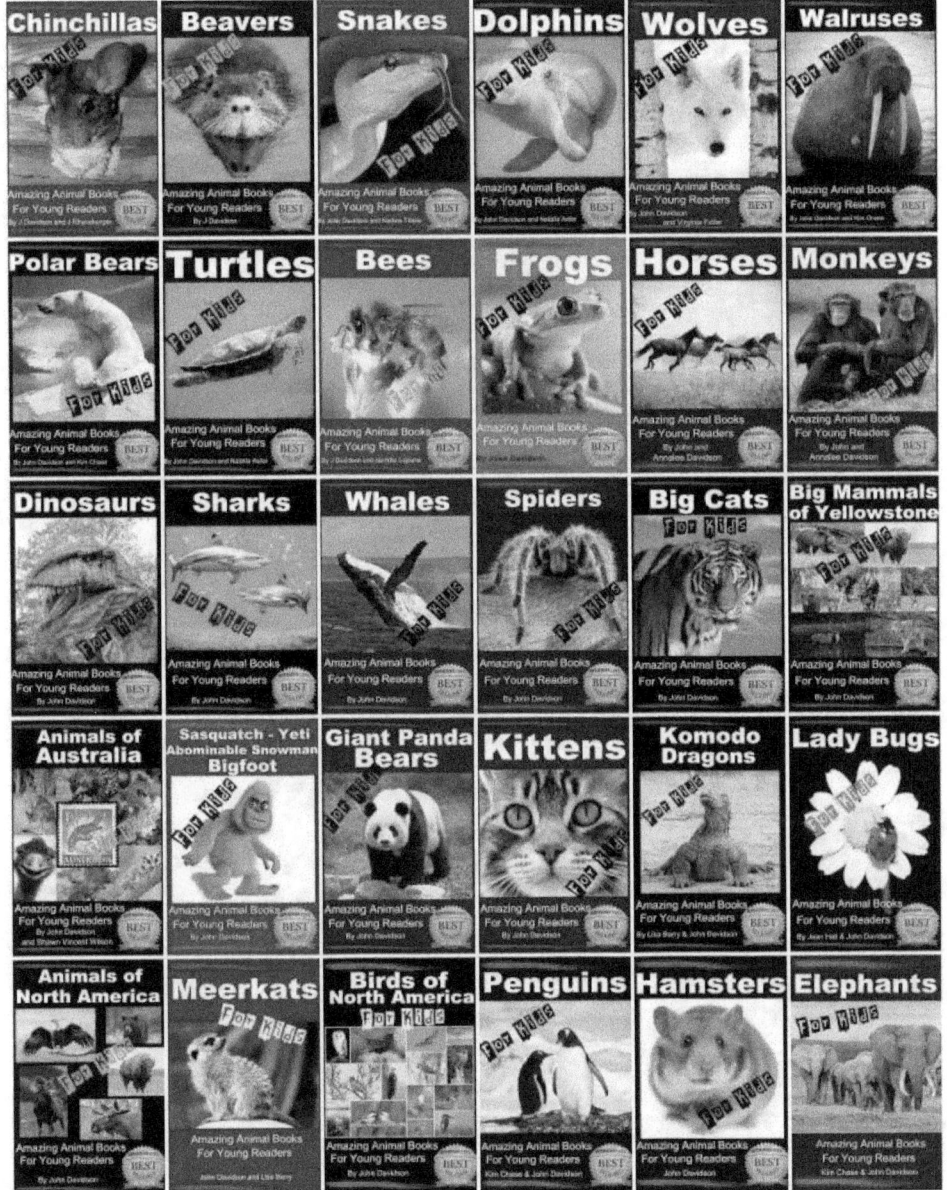

Staying Healthy – Tips and Techniques For Heart Patients

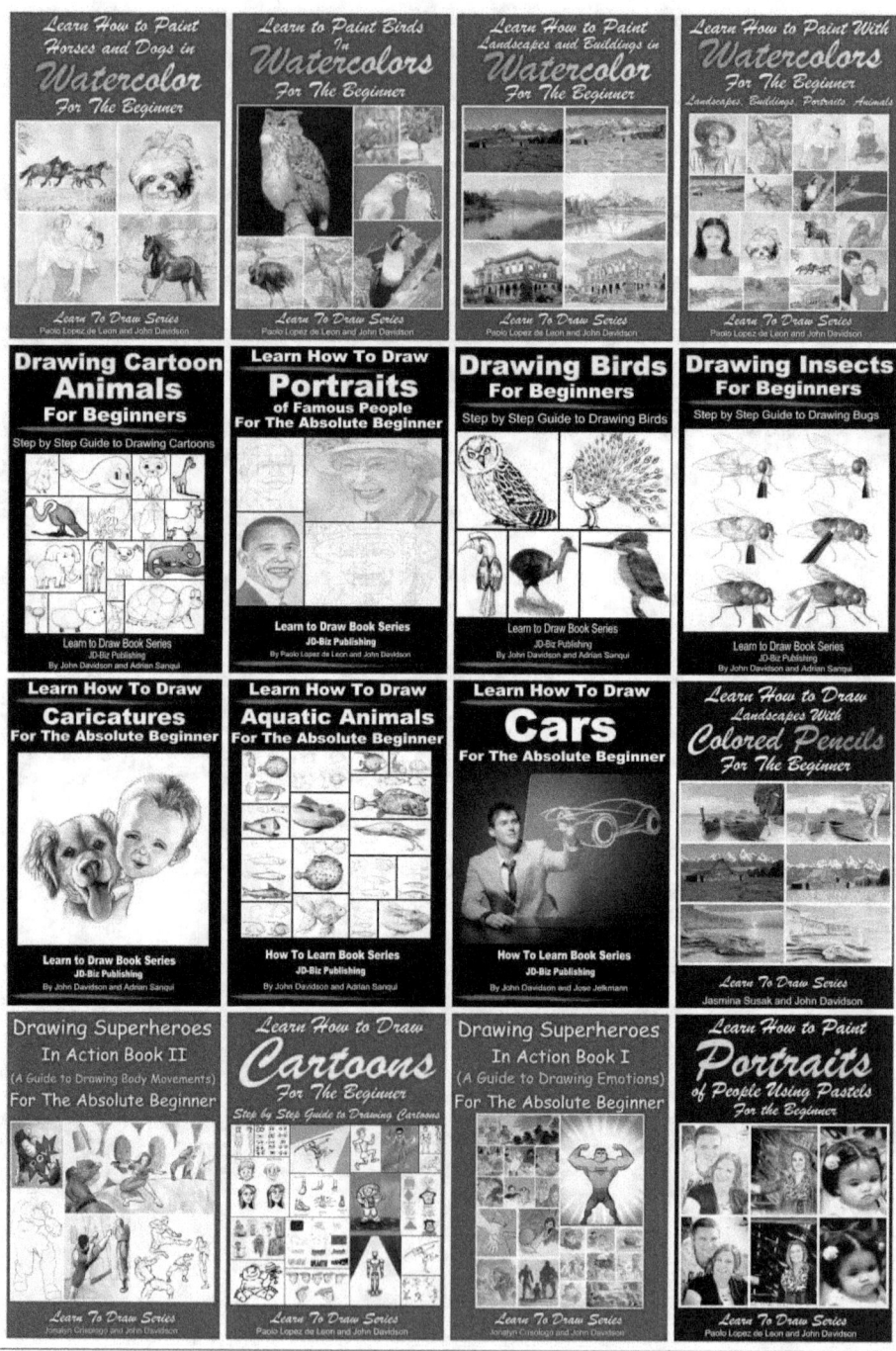

Staying Healthy – Tips and Techniques For Heart Patients

How to Build and Plan Books

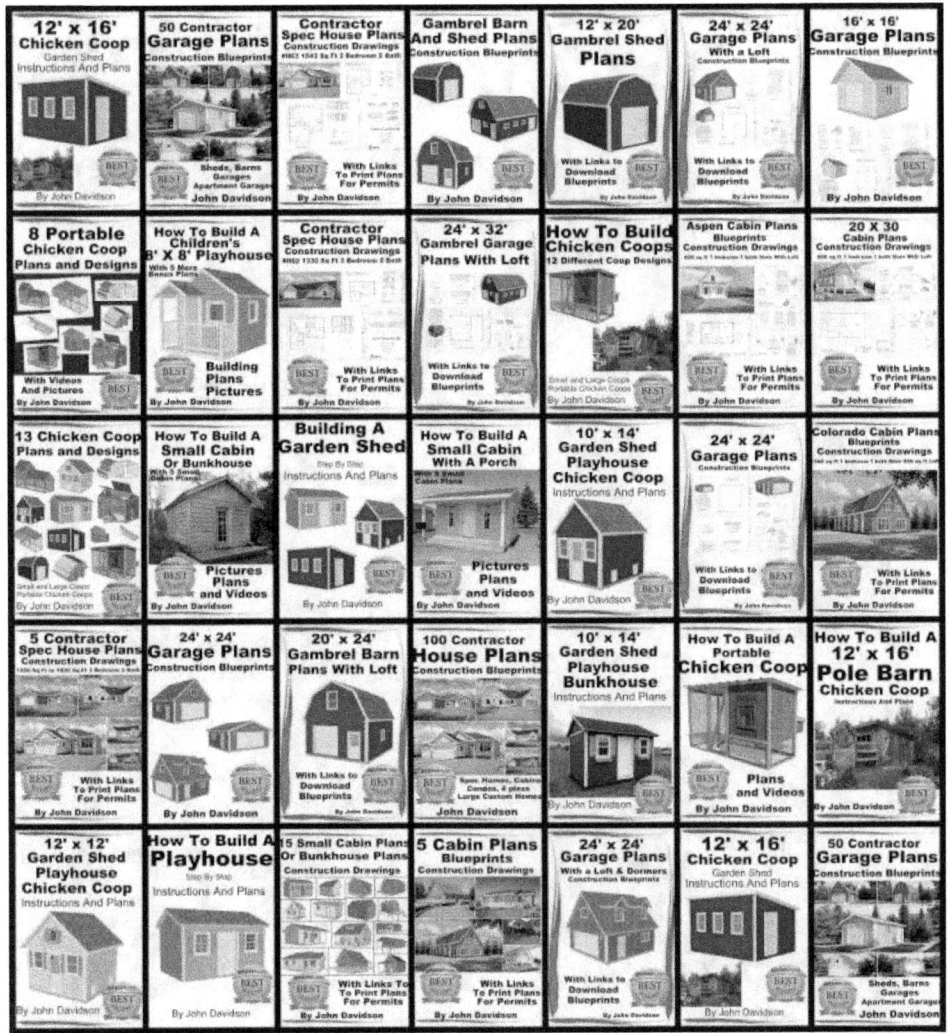

Staying Healthy – Tips and Techniques For Heart Patients

Entrepreneur Book Series

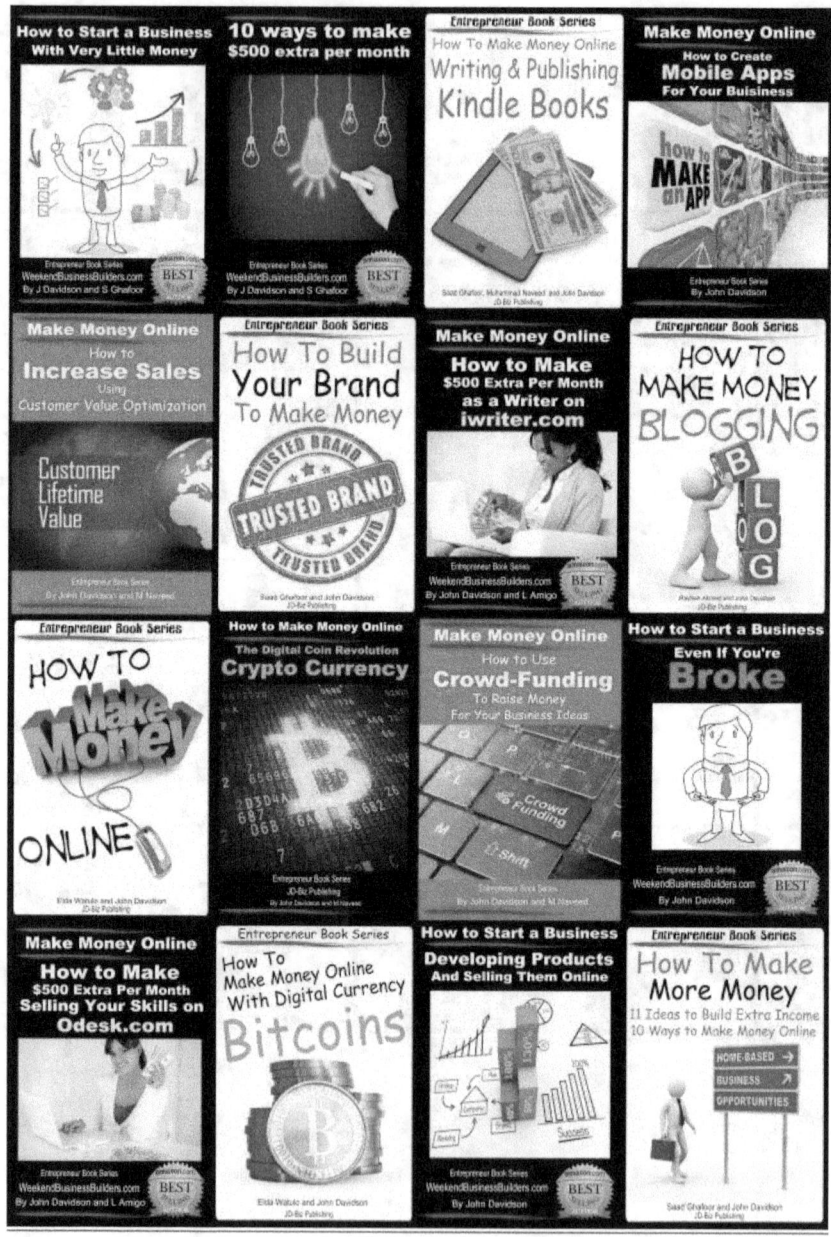

Staying Healthy – Tips and Techniques For Heart Patients

Publisher

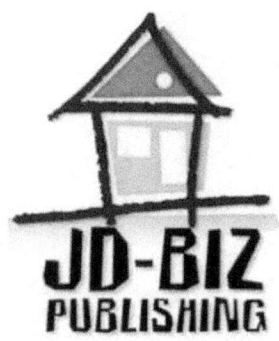

JD-Biz Corp

P O Box 374

Mendon, Utah 84325

http://www.jd-biz.com/

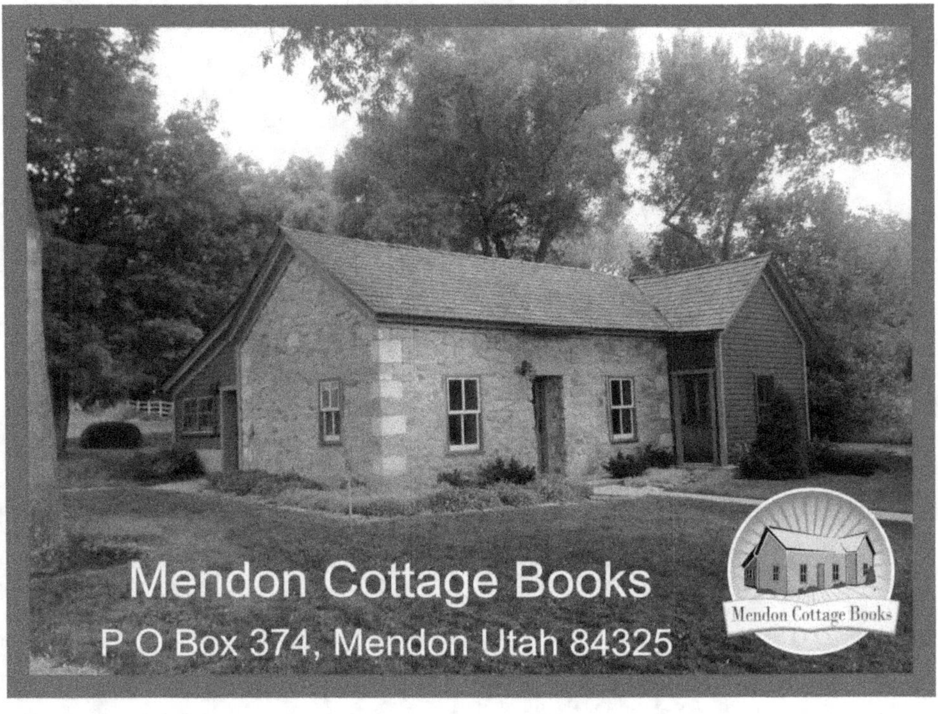

Mendon Cottage Books

P O Box 374, Mendon Utah 84325

Staying Healthy – Tips and Techniques For Heart Patients

www.ingramcontent.com/pod-product-compliance
Lightning Source LLC
Chambersburg PA
CBHW061929280526
45787CB00004B/1534